# SOMATIC EXERCISES FOR BEGINNERS

## Carefully Curated Guide to Help Relieve Tension, Eliminate Anxiety, and Live a fulfilling Life

By

VANESSA H. GOURDINE

# TABLE OF CONTENTS

# INTRODUCTION

Imagine waking up every morning feeling stiff, your body weighed down by tension and aches that seem to have no clear origin. You've tried stretching, conventional exercises, maybe even some yoga, but nothing seems to provide lasting relief. The tightness returns, your range of motion remains limited, and with each passing day, the frustration builds. It feels like you're trapped in your own body, desperate for a way out but unsure where to turn.

This was Sarah's life. A busy professional in her early forties, Sarah had always prided herself on staying active. Yet, despite her efforts, she found herself increasingly plagued by discomfort that disrupted her daily routine and left her feeling disconnected from her body. No matter how much she stretched or strengthened her muscles, the tension persisted, sapping her energy and affecting her quality of life.

One day, a friend introduced Sarah to somatic exercises, a practice she had never heard of before. Intrigued but skeptical, Sarah decided to give it a try. What did she have to lose? Little did she know, this decision would change everything.

As she began to explore somatic movements, Sarah discovered a profound connection between her mind and body that she had never experienced before. The exercises were gentle, yet their impact was immediate. She felt her muscles releasing, her posture improving, and her mind calming. For the first time in years, Sarah felt truly at ease in her own body. The tension that had once seemed inescapable began to melt away, replaced by a newfound sense of freedom and ease.

Sarah's story is not unique. Many people, perhaps even you, struggle with chronic tension, pain, or a lack of flexibility that conventional methods just can't seem to address. If you've ever felt stuck in a cycle of discomfort, wondering why nothing seems to work, then this book is for you.

**"Somatic Exercises for Beginners"** is designed to guide you on a journey of self-discovery and healing, offering a gentle yet powerful approach to reconnecting with your body. In these pages, you'll learn how to move with intention, listen to the signals your body sends, and unlock the natural capacity for self-healing that lies within you.

Whether you're dealing with chronic pain, seeking to improve your flexibility and strength, or simply looking for a way to relieve stress and find balance, this book provides the tools and techniques you need. Through a blend of somatic exercises and carefully selected yoga poses, you'll discover a practice that is not only accessible but also transformative.

Say goodbye to the frustration of fleeting relief and hello to a lasting solution. By embracing somatic exercises, you can reclaim your body, restore your sense of ease, and step into a life of greater vitality and well-being.

Let's begin this journey together—your body is waiting to be rediscovered.

# SECTION I

# CHAPTER 1

# WHAT ARE SOMATIC EXERCISES?

Somatic exercises are a form of movement practice that focuses on increasing body awareness, improving mobility, and reducing chronic tension by reconnecting the mind with the body. Unlike traditional exercise routines that often emphasise external goals like muscle strengthening or cardiovascular fitness, somatic exercises delve into the internal experience of movement. The word "somatic" comes from the Greek word "soma," meaning "body," but in this context, it refers to the body as perceived from within.

Somatic exercises involve slow, mindful movements designed to help you become aware of habitual movement patterns and release chronic muscle tension. By paying close attention to how your body moves and feels during these exercises, you can retrain your nervous system, develop a deeper understanding of your physical self, and enhance your overall well-being. These exercises are often gentle, making them accessible to people of all ages and fitness levels.

Somatic practices have roots in various disciplines, including the Feldenkrais Method, Alexander Technique, and Hanna Somatics, each offering a unique approach to exploring the body-mind connection. Whether you're looking to relieve pain, improve flexibility, or simply reconnect with your body, somatic exercises offer a path to greater self-awareness and physical freedom.

## The Science Behind Somatic Movement

The effectiveness of somatic exercises lies in their ability to tap into the nervous system and rewire habitual movement patterns that contribute to chronic pain and tension. The human body is designed to move fluidly and efficiently, but over time, factors like injury, stress, poor posture, and repetitive movements can lead to the development of unconscious muscle contractions and dysfunctional movement patterns.

These patterns become deeply ingrained in the brain's motor cortex, leading to what is known as "sensory-motor amnesia."

Sensory-motor amnesia occurs when the brain loses the ability to fully control certain muscles, causing them to remain in a state of partial contraction even when at rest. This can result in chronic pain, stiffness, and limited range of motion. Somatic exercises work by bringing these unconscious patterns into conscious awareness, allowing the brain to "reset" and restore normal muscle function.

When you perform a somatic exercise, you are engaging in a process called "pandiculation," which involves three steps: contracting a muscle group, slowly releasing the contraction, and then fully relaxing the muscles. This process sends a signal to the brain that helps it regain voluntary control over the muscles, effectively reprogramming the nervous system to break free from habitual tension.

Research in neuroscience supports the effectiveness of somatic exercises. Studies have shown that mindful movement practices can enhance proprioception (the body's sense of its position in space), improve motor control, and reduce pain by altering the way the brain perceives and responds to the body's signals. By retraining the brain and nervous system, somatic exercises can lead to long-lasting improvements in movement quality and overall physical health.

## Benefits of Somatic Exercises

Somatic exercises offer a wide range of benefits that go beyond physical fitness. Here are some of the key advantages:

1. **Pain Relief**: One of the most significant benefits of somatic exercises is their

ability to alleviate chronic pain. By addressing the root cause of pain—sensory-motor amnesia—somatic exercises can help release tension and restore normal muscle function, providing relief from conditions such as back pain, neck pain, and joint discomfort.

2. **Improved Flexibility and Mobility**: Somatic exercises gently stretch and lengthen muscles, improving flexibility and range of motion. Unlike static stretching, which can sometimes exacerbate muscle tension, somatic exercises encourage fluid, natural movement patterns that enhance overall mobility.

3. **Increased Body Awareness**: By practicing somatic exercises, you develop a heightened sense of body awareness,

which allows you to recognize and correct dysfunctional movement patterns. This increased awareness can help prevent injuries, improve posture, and enhance your overall physical performance.

4. **Stress Reduction**: Somatic exercises incorporate mindful movement and deep breathing, which help to calm the nervous system and reduce stress. The practice encourages relaxation and a sense of ease, making it an effective tool for managing anxiety and tension.

5. **Enhanced Coordination and Balance**: Through the practice of somatic exercises, you can improve your coordination and balance by refining your body's ability to move efficiently and smoothly. This is particularly beneficial for older adults or individuals recovering from injury.

6. **Better Posture**: Many people suffer from poor posture due to prolonged sitting, repetitive tasks, or stress. Somatic exercises help to realign the body, releasing tension in areas like the shoulders, neck, and lower back, which in turn improves posture.

7. **Emotional Well-being**: The mind-body connection fostered by somatic exercises can also positively impact your emotional health. As you become more in tune with your body, you may find that emotional tensions are also released, leading to a greater sense of inner peace and well-being.

## Who Can Benefit from This Book?

**"Somatic Exercises for Beginners"** is designed for anyone who is interested in improving their physical and mental well-being through mindful movement. Whether you're a complete novice to exercise or someone with years of experience, this book offers something valuable for everyone. Here are some of the groups who will benefit most:

1. **Individuals Experiencing Chronic Pain**: If you're struggling with chronic pain or discomfort, somatic exercises can offer a gentle yet effective solution. This book provides you with the tools to alleviate pain by addressing its root causes, helping you regain control over your body and reduce reliance on pain medications.

2. **Those Looking to Improve Flexibility and Mobility**: This book is ideal for anyone who wants to enhance their flexibility and mobility. The exercises within are designed to help you move more freely and with greater ease, making everyday activities more enjoyable.

3. **People Under Stress or Anxiety**: If you're feeling overwhelmed by stress or anxiety, the somatic exercises in this book can help you find relief. By focusing on the mind-body connection and practicing mindful movement, you can reduce tension and cultivate a sense of calm.

4. **Older Adults Seeking Gentle Exercise**: Somatic exercises are particularly well-suited for older adults, as they are low-impact and gentle on the body. This book provides a safe and accessible way

for seniors to stay active, improve balance, and maintain independence.

5. **Athletes and Fitness Enthusiasts**: Even if you're already active, somatic exercises can complement your existing routine by helping you refine your movement patterns, prevent injuries, and improve overall performance.

6. **Rehabilitation Patients**: For those recovering from injury or surgery, somatic exercises offer a gentle way to regain strength, flexibility, and coordination. This book provides a step-by-step guide to help you safely ease back into movement.

7. **Anyone Curious About the Mind-Body Connection**: If you're intrigued by the concept of the mind-body connection and want to explore it further, this book will guide you through the principles of

somatic movement and help you discover the profound impact it can have on your life.

No matter your background or fitness level, **"Somatic Exercises for Beginners"** is a comprehensive guide that will empower you to take control of your physical and emotional health. By incorporating these exercises into your daily routine, you can experience greater ease in your body, a clearer mind, and a more fulfilling life.

# CHAPTER 2

# UNDERSTANDING SOMATICS

Somatic practices offer a unique approach to movement and healing, focusing on the integration of mind and body to improve physical and mental well-being. Unlike traditional exercise routines that emphasize external outcomes, such as muscle growth or cardiovascular endurance, somatic practices prioritize internal awareness and the ability to consciously control the body. This focus on self-perception and mindful movement can lead to profound changes in how we move, feel, and interact with our environment. To truly appreciate the value of somatic exercises, it's essential to understand their origins, key principles, and how they differ from traditional workouts.

## The Origins of Somatic Practices

The concept of "somatics" derives from the Greek word "soma," meaning "body," but in somatic practice, it refers to the body as it is experienced from within. This internal perspective is at the heart of somatic practices, which aim to reconnect individuals with their own bodies, allowing them to feel and move more freely and naturally.

The origins of somatic practices can be traced back to the early 20th century when pioneers in movement and bodywork began to explore new ways of understanding and experiencing the body. One of the most influential figures in the development of somatic practices was Thomas Hanna, who coined the term "somatics" in the 1970s. Hanna's work was heavily influenced by earlier pioneers such as F. Matthias Alexander, Moshe Feldenkrais, and Elsa Gindler, who each contributed unique perspectives to the field.

F. Matthias Alexander, an Australian actor turned educator, developed the Alexander Technique in the late 19th and early 20th centuries. Alexander's approach emphasized the importance of body alignment and posture, particularly in relation to the head, neck, and spine. He discovered that many of the physical problems people experienced were due to unconscious habits that interfered with natural movement. The Alexander Technique focuses on bringing these habits into conscious awareness and retraining the body to move more efficiently and comfortably.

Moshe Feldenkrais, an Israeli engineer, physicist, and judo expert, further advanced the field of somatics with the development of the Feldenkrais Method. Feldenkrais, who suffered from chronic knee pain, began exploring alternative methods of movement and healing. He believed that the brain's plasticity allowed for the retraining of movement patterns, even in cases of injury or dysfunction. The Feldenkrais Method uses gentle, exploratory movements to increase body awareness and improve movement efficiency.

Elsa Gindler, a German teacher and somatic educator, developed a method of bodywork that focused on the relationship between movement, breath, and awareness. Gindler's work, which she called "Unmittelbare Leibesübungen" (direct body exercises), emphasized the importance of experiencing the body from within and cultivating a deep sense of presence in movement. Her approach influenced many subsequent somatic educators, including Charlotte Selver, who brought Gindler's work to the United States and developed it into the practice known as Sensory Awareness.

Thomas Hanna, building on the work of these pioneers, developed Hanna Somatics, a method that focuses on addressing chronic pain and dysfunction through conscious movement. Hanna introduced the concept of "sensory-motor amnesia," a condition in which the brain loses the ability to fully control certain muscles due to habitual patterns of tension and contraction. Hanna Somatics aims to reverse sensory-motor amnesia by bringing unconscious movement patterns into conscious awareness and retraining the nervous system to restore natural, pain-free movement.

Together, these pioneers laid the foundation for modern somatic practices, each contributing unique insights into the relationship between the mind and body. Their work continues to influence a wide range of somatic practices today, from movement therapy and bodywork to yoga and mindfulness meditation.

## Key Principles of Somatic Movement

Somatic movement is grounded in several key principles that differentiate it from other forms of exercise and physical therapy. These principles emphasise the importance of internal awareness, conscious control, and the holistic integration of mind and body.

1. **Body Awareness**: The cornerstone of somatic practices is the development of body awareness, or the ability to perceive and feel the body from within. This involves paying close attention to the sensations, movements, and positions of the body, often with a focus on specific areas of tension or discomfort. By cultivating body awareness, individuals can become more attuned to their habitual movement patterns and learn to identify areas of restriction or imbalance.

2. **Mindful Movement**: Somatic exercises are performed slowly and mindfully, with an emphasis on exploring the quality of movement rather than achieving specific

physical goals. This mindful approach allows individuals to notice subtle changes in their body and movement patterns, leading to greater control and precision in their movements. Mindful movement also encourages a sense of presence and relaxation, which can help reduce stress and tension.

3. **Self-Regulation**: Somatic practices empower individuals to take an active role in their own healing and well-being. Rather than relying on external interventions, such as medication or surgery, somatic exercises teach individuals to listen to their bodies and make conscious choices about how they move and respond to their environment. This self-regulation fosters a sense of autonomy and self-efficacy, which can be

particularly empowering for those dealing with chronic pain or injury.

4. **Neuroplasticity**: A key principle of somatic movement is the idea that the brain and nervous system are capable of change, even in adulthood. This concept, known as neuroplasticity, suggests that habitual movement patterns can be retrained, and new, more efficient patterns can be established. Somatic exercises leverage neuroplasticity by encouraging the brain to create new neural pathways that support healthy, pain-free movement.

5. **Holistic Integration**: Somatic practices view the body as a holistic, interconnected system in which all parts work together to support overall well-being. This perspective emphasizes the importance of integrating physical, mental, and

emotional aspects of the self. By addressing the body as a whole, rather than focusing on isolated symptoms or areas of dysfunction, somatic exercises promote overall health and vitality.

6. **Gentle Exploration**: Unlike traditional workouts that often push the body to its limits, somatic exercises are gentle and exploratory. This approach allows individuals to move within their comfort zone, gradually expanding their range of motion and improving movement quality without causing strain or injury. The emphasis is on discovering new ways of moving that feel natural and effortless.

These principles form the foundation of somatic movement practices and guide the way in which exercises are performed and experienced. By embracing these principles, individuals can develop a deeper connection with their bodies and achieve greater physical and emotional well-being.

## How Somatic Exercises Differ from Traditional Workouts

Somatic exercises differ significantly from traditional workouts in both their goals and methods. While traditional exercise routines often focus on external objectives, such as building muscle strength, increasing cardiovascular endurance, or losing weight, somatic exercises prioritise internal awareness and the quality of movement. This fundamental difference leads to a variety of distinctions in how somatic exercises are practised and experienced.

1. **Focus on Internal Awareness**: In traditional workouts, the emphasis is often on external outcomes, such as lifting a certain amount of weight, running a specific distance, or achieving a particular body shape. Somatic exercises, on the other hand, focus on developing internal awareness and sensitivity to the body's sensations and movements. The goal is not to achieve a specific physical result but to improve the way the body feels and moves from within.

2. **Mind-Body Integration**: Traditional workouts often separate the mind and body, with the body being treated as a machine to be trained or conditioned. In contrast, somatic exercises emphasize the integration of mind and body, recognizing that thoughts, emotions, and physical

sensations are interconnected and influence one another. This holistic approach encourages individuals to move with intention and awareness, leading to more balanced and harmonious movement.

3. **Gentle and Slow Movements**: Traditional exercise routines often involve high-intensity movements, heavy lifting, or repetitive motions performed at a fast pace. Somatic exercises, however, are characterised by gentle, slow, and deliberate movements. This slower pace allows individuals to pay close attention to the sensations in their body, making it easier to notice and correct dysfunctional movement patterns. The emphasis is on quality of movement rather than quantity.

4. **Emphasis on Functionality**: While traditional workouts often focus on specific muscle groups or fitness goals, somatic exercises prioritize functional movement patterns that are relevant to everyday activities. The goal is to improve overall movement efficiency, coordination, and ease, making it easier to perform daily tasks without pain or discomfort. This functional approach is particularly beneficial for individuals recovering from injury or dealing with chronic pain.

5. **Self-Directed Learning**: In traditional workouts, individuals often rely on external cues from instructors, trainers, or equipment to guide their movements. Somatic exercises, however, encourage self-directed learning, where individuals

are invited to explore their own movement patterns and discover what feels best for their bodies. This self-directed approach fosters a sense of curiosity and experimentation, allowing individuals to find solutions that work specifically for them.

6. **Therapeutic Focus**: While traditional workouts are often geared towards achieving physical fitness, somatic exercises have a therapeutic focus, addressing underlying issues such as chronic pain, tension, or movement dysfunction. By targeting the root causes of these issues, somatic exercises can lead to lasting improvements in physical and emotional well-being.

7. **Non-Competitive Approach**: Traditional workouts can sometimes foster a

competitive mindset, where individuals are encouraged to push themselves to outperform others or achieve personal bests. Somatic exercises, however, adopt a non-competitive approach, where the focus is on individual exploration and self-discovery. The goal is to move in a way that feels comfortable and sustainable, without the pressure to meet external standards or compete with others.

# CHAPTER 3

# PREPARING FOR YOUR SOMATIC JOURNEY

Embarking on a somatic journey is a transformative experience that goes beyond traditional exercise routines. It involves a deep connection between the mind and body, emphasizing internal awareness, mindful movement, and holistic well-being. Preparing for this journey requires more than just physical readiness; it involves a thoughtful approach to understanding your body's needs, setting achievable goals, creating an environment conducive to practice, and equipping yourself with the right tools and techniques. This comprehensive guide will help you prepare for your somatic journey, ensuring that you start with the right mindset and foundation.

**Assessing Your Body's Needs**

Before beginning your somatic practice, it's essential to take a moment to assess your body's current state and needs. Understanding where you are physically and emotionally will help you tailor your practice to address specific concerns and goals. Here's how you can assess your body's needs:

1. **Physical Condition**: Start by evaluating your overall physical condition. Consider any areas of chronic pain, stiffness, or discomfort. Are there specific movements or activities that cause you discomfort?

Identifying these areas will help you focus on exercises that can relieve tension and improve mobility.

2. **Movement Patterns**: Pay attention to your habitual movement patterns. How do you sit, stand, walk, or perform daily activities? Notice if there are any imbalances, asymmetries, or restrictions in your movements. Somatic exercises often address these habitual patterns, helping to retrain your body for more efficient and comfortable movement.

3. **Body Awareness**: Assess your level of body awareness. How in tune are you with your body's sensations? Do you notice subtle cues of tension, relaxation, or alignment? Developing body awareness is a key component of somatic practice, and starting with an understanding of your

current awareness level will guide your progress.

4. **Emotional State**: Consider your emotional state and how it affects your body. Stress, anxiety, and other emotional factors can manifest as physical tension or discomfort. Understanding the connection between your emotions and physical sensations will help you approach your practice holistically.

5. **Previous Injuries or Conditions**: Take into account any previous injuries, surgeries, or medical conditions that may impact your movement. It's important to approach somatic exercises with care, especially if you have any limitations or contraindications. Consult with a healthcare professional if you have any

concerns about starting a new movement practice.

By taking the time to assess your body's needs, you'll be better equipped to choose the right somatic exercises and tailor your practice to your unique situation. This self-assessment also helps you set realistic goals for your journey.

**Setting Realistic Goals**

Setting realistic and achievable goals is an essential part of preparing for your somatic journey. Goals provide direction and motivation, helping you stay focused and committed to your practice. However, it's important to set goals that are both challenging and attainable to avoid frustration or burnout.

1. **Start Small**: Begin by setting small, manageable goals that align with your

current abilities and needs. For example, if you're dealing with chronic pain, a goal might be to reduce discomfort in a specific area, such as your lower back, through daily somatic exercises. Starting with smaller goals allows you to build confidence and track your progress over time.

2. **Focus on Process Over Outcome**: In somatic practice, the journey is just as important as the destination. Rather than focusing solely on the outcome (e.g., achieving a certain level of flexibility or pain relief), emphasize the process of becoming more aware of your body and improving your movement quality. This approach encourages mindfulness and reduces the pressure to achieve specific results quickly.

3. **Be Flexible**: Recognize that your goals may evolve as you progress in your somatic journey. Be open to adjusting your goals based on how your body responds to the practice. Flexibility in goal-setting allows you to adapt to new challenges and discoveries along the way.

4. **Set Both Short-Term and Long-Term Goals**: Establish a mix of short-term and long-term goals. Short-term goals provide immediate motivation and satisfaction, while long-term goals give you something to work toward over an extended period. For instance, a short-term goal might be to improve your posture, while a long-term goal could be to increase overall mobility and reduce chronic pain.

5. **Celebrate Progress**: Acknowledge and celebrate your progress, no matter how

small. Recognizing your achievements, whether it's increased body awareness or reduced tension in a particular area, reinforces positive behavior and keeps you motivated.

By setting realistic goals, you create a clear path for your somatic journey, allowing you to progress at your own pace and achieve meaningful results.

**Creating a Comfortable Practice Space**

The environment in which you practice somatic exercises plays a significant role in your overall experience. A comfortable, peaceful, and inviting space can enhance your focus, relaxation, and body awareness. Here's how to create an ideal practice space:

1. **Choose a Quiet Location**: Find a space in your home or environment where you can practice without distractions. A quiet location helps you focus on your movements and sensations, allowing for deeper connection with your body. If possible, choose a space with minimal noise and interruptions.

2. **Ensure Adequate Space**: Make sure your practice area has enough room for you to move freely without feeling cramped. You'll need space to stretch, lie down, and perform various movements comfortably. Clear any clutter or obstacles that could hinder your practice.

3. **Control Lighting**: The lighting in your practice space can affect your mood and concentration. Soft, natural lighting is ideal, as it creates a calming atmosphere.

If natural light isn't available, consider using dimmable lamps or candles to create a warm, soothing ambiance.

4. **Use Comfortable Flooring**: Somatic exercises often involve lying on the floor, so it's important to have a comfortable surface to practice on. A yoga mat, carpet, or padded floor covering can provide cushioning and support. Ensure that the surface is clean and free of any sharp objects or debris.

5. **Incorporate Relaxing Elements**: Enhance your practice space with elements that promote relaxation and mindfulness. This could include items like essential oil diffusers, calming music, plants, or inspirational artwork. These elements can help create a positive and peaceful environment for your practice.

6. **Maintain a Consistent Practice Space**: If possible, designate a specific area for your somatic practice and use it consistently. Having a dedicated practice space helps establish a routine and signals to your mind and body that it's time to focus on your well-being.

By creating a comfortable and inviting practice space, you set the stage for a successful somatic journey. A well-prepared environment supports your physical and mental relaxation, allowing you to fully engage in your practice.

## Essential Equipment and Attire

While somatic exercises are generally low-tech and require minimal equipment, having the right tools and attire can enhance your practice and make it more enjoyable. Here's what you'll need:

1. **Yoga Mat**: A yoga mat is a versatile piece of equipment that provides cushioning and support for floor-based exercises. It helps prevent slipping and offers a comfortable surface for lying, sitting, and kneeling movements. Choose a mat with adequate thickness and grip to suit your needs.

2. **Bolsters and Cushions**: Bolsters and cushions can be used to support various parts of your body during somatic exercises. They help you maintain proper alignment and reduce strain on joints and muscles. These props are especially useful for individuals with limited flexibility or those recovering from injury.

3. **Blankets**: A blanket can be used for additional padding or warmth during your practice. It can also be folded or rolled to create support for specific exercises. Having a blanket on hand allows you to adapt your practice to different levels of comfort.

4. **Comfortable Clothing**: Wear loose, comfortable clothing that allows you to move freely. Avoid tight or restrictive garments that could limit your range of motion or cause discomfort. Breathable, stretchy fabrics like cotton or moisture-wicking materials are ideal for somatic practice.

5. **Pillows**: Pillows can be used to support your head, neck, or lower back during certain exercises. They provide extra

comfort and help you maintain proper posture throughout your practice.

6. **Water Bottle**: Staying hydrated is important during any form of exercise, including somatic practice. Keep a water bottle nearby to sip on as needed, especially if your practice includes breathwork or more vigorous movements.

7. **Timer or Clock**: A timer or clock can help you keep track of the duration of your practice or specific exercises. Setting a timer for certain exercises allows you to focus on the quality of movement without constantly checking the time.

8. **Journal or Notebook**: Consider keeping a journal or notebook to record your experiences, observations, and progress. Reflecting on your practice can deepen

your understanding of your body and help you track changes over time.

By having the essential equipment and attire ready, you'll be well-prepared to engage in your somatic journey comfortably and effectively.

**Breathing Techniques for Somatic Practice**

Breathing is a fundamental aspect of somatic practice, as it directly influences your body's tension, relaxation, and overall movement quality. Proper breathing techniques can enhance your practice by promoting relaxation, increasing body awareness, and supporting mindful movement. Here are some key breathing techniques to incorporate into your somatic exercises:

1. **Diaphragmatic Breathing**: Also known as belly breathing, diaphragmatic

breathing involves deep breaths that fill your lungs and expand your diaphragm. This technique encourages full oxygen exchange, reduces tension, and promotes relaxation. To practice diaphragmatic breathing:

- Lie on your back or sit comfortably with your spine straight.
- Place one hand on your chest and the other on your abdomen.
- Inhale deeply through your nose, allowing your abdomen to rise while keeping your chest relatively still.
- Exhale slowly through your mouth, feeling your abdomen fall.
- Repeat for several breaths, focusing on the sensation of your breath moving in and out of your body.

2. **4-7-8 Breathing**: This calming breath technique, developed by Dr. Andrew Weil, is designed to reduce stress and anxiety by regulating your breath. The 4-7-8 pattern helps you focus your mind and relax your body. To practice 4-7-8 breathing:
   - Inhale quietly through your nose for a count of four.
   - Hold your breath for a count of seven.
   - Exhale completely through your mouth for a count of eight, making a whooshing sound.
   - Repeat the cycle for three to four rounds, gradually increasing the number of cycles as you become more comfortable.

3. **Alternate Nostril Breathing**: Alternate nostril breathing, or Nadi Shodhana, is a yoga breathing technique that balances the nervous system and promotes mental clarity. This technique involves breathing through one nostril at a time while blocking the other. To practice alternate nostril breathing:

- Sit comfortably with your spine straight and shoulders relaxed.
- Close your right nostril with your right thumb.
- Inhale deeply through your left nostril.
- Close your left nostril with your right ring finger, release your right nostril, and exhale through the right nostril.

- o Inhale through the right nostril, close it with your thumb, release the left nostril, and exhale through the left nostril.
  - o Continue alternating nostrils for several breaths, focusing on the flow of breath and the calming effect it has on your mind and body.

4. **Box Breathing**: Box breathing, also known as square breathing, is a simple and effective technique for grounding and centering your mind. It involves breathing in a square pattern, with equal counts for inhaling, holding, exhaling, and holding. To practice box breathing:
   - o Inhale through your nose for a count of four.
   - o Hold your breath for a count of four.

- Exhale through your mouth for a count of four.
- Hold your breath for a count of four.
- Repeat the cycle for several rounds, visualizing a square as you breathe.

5. **Ocean Breath (Ujjayi Pranayama)**: Ujjayi breath, or ocean breath, is a yoga technique that creates a soothing sound similar to ocean waves. This breath is often used during yoga practice to maintain a steady rhythm and focus. To practice ocean breath:

   - Inhale deeply through your nose.
   - As you exhale, slightly constrict the back of your throat, creating a soft hissing or ocean-like sound.

- Continue breathing in and out through your nose with this constriction, maintaining a steady and rhythmic breath.
- Focus on the sound and sensation of your breath as it moves in and out of your body.

Incorporating these breathing techniques into your somatic practice enhances your ability to connect with your body, regulate your nervous system, and deepen your overall experience. Breathing is not just an auxiliary component; it is integral to the mindful and holistic nature of somatic exercises.

Preparing for your somatic journey involves more than just understanding the exercises themselves. It requires a thoughtful approach to assessing your body's needs, setting realistic goals, creating a comfortable practice space, equipping yourself with essential tools, and mastering breathing techniques. By taking these steps, you lay a strong foundation for a transformative experience that promotes mind-body integration, movement efficiency, and overall well-being. As you embark on this journey, remember that somatic practice is a personal and evolving process—one that will continually deepen your connection with your body and enhance your quality of life.

# SECTION II

# CHAPTER 4

# SOMATIC EXERCISES FOR FLEXIBILITY

**1.** *Pelvic Tilt*

**Target Areas:** Lower back, hips, and pelvic region

**Benefits:** Improves lower back flexibility, reduces tension in the pelvic area, and enhances spinal mobility.

**Instructions:**

1. **Starting Position:** Lie on your back with your knees bent and feet flat on the floor, hip-width apart. Arms should rest comfortably by your sides.

2. **Engage Your Core:** Take a deep breath in, and as you exhale, gently engage your abdominal muscles. This will help to stabilize your core.

3. **Tilt the Pelvis:** Inhale deeply. As you exhale, gently flatten your lower back against the floor by tilting your pelvis backward (posterior tilt). This action should bring your pubic bone closer to your navel.

4. **Hold and Release:** Hold this position for a few seconds while continuing to breathe normally. Inhale as you slowly return to the neutral position (where there is a natural curve in your lower back).

5. **Repetition:** Repeat this movement 8-10 times, focusing on the smoothness and control of the movement.

## 2. *Cat-Cow Stretch*

**Target Areas:** Spine, shoulders, neck

**Benefits:** Increases spinal flexibility, stretches the back and neck muscles, and improves posture.

**Instructions:**

1. **Starting Position:** Begin on your hands and knees in a tabletop position. Your wrists should be directly under your shoulders, and your knees under your hips.

2. **Cat Pose (Flexion):** Inhale deeply, and as you exhale, round your spine toward the

ceiling (like a scared cat). Tuck your chin toward your chest, and draw your navel in toward your spine.

3. **Cow Pose (Extension):** Inhale as you reverse the motion, allowing your belly to drop toward the floor, arching your back. Lift your head and tailbone toward the ceiling, opening your chest.

4. **Flow Between Poses:** Continue to alternate between Cat and Cow poses with each inhale and exhale, moving smoothly and mindfully.

5. **Repetition:** Perform 10-12 cycles, focusing on the flexibility and fluidity of the spine.

### 3. *Somatic Neck Release*

**Target Areas:** Neck, shoulders

**Benefits:** Releases tension in the neck, improves flexibility, and promotes relaxation.

**Instructions:**

1. **Starting Position:** Sit or stand comfortably with your spine straight and shoulders relaxed.

2. **Neck Stretch:** Slowly drop your right ear toward your right shoulder. Hold this position and take a few deep breaths, feeling the stretch on the left side of your neck.

3. **Explore Movement:** Gently nod your head up and down, as if saying "yes," while maintaining the side bend. Notice

how the stretch changes in different parts of the neck.

4. **Return and Repeat:** Slowly bring your head back to the center, and then repeat on the left side, dropping your left ear toward your left shoulder.

5. **Repetition:** Perform 3-5 stretches on each side, taking your time to explore the sensations in your neck.

### 4. *Hamstring Release*

**Target Areas:** Hamstrings, lower back

**Benefits:** Lengthens the hamstrings, reduces lower back tension, and enhances flexibility in the posterior chain.

**Instructions:**

1. **Starting Position:** Lie on your back with your knees bent and feet flat on the floor.

2. **Raise One Leg:** Slowly extend your right leg toward the ceiling, keeping your knee slightly bent. Hold the back of your thigh with both hands.

3. **Flex and Point:** Gently flex your foot (toes pointing toward you) to deepen the stretch in your hamstring. Hold for a few breaths, then point your toes to release the stretch.

4. **Dynamic Movement:** Slowly lower and lift your leg while keeping your hands on your thigh, exploring the range of motion in your hamstring.

5. **Repeat on the Other Side:** After several repetitions, switch to the left leg and repeat the sequence.

6. **Repetition:** Perform 5-8 repetitions on each side.

## 5. *Side-Lying Hip Release*

**Target Areas:** Hips, glutes

**Benefits:** Increases hip flexibility, reduces tension in the glutes, and improves hip mobility.

## Instructions:

1. **Starting Position:** Lie on your left side with your legs stacked and knees bent at a 90-degree angle. Rest your head on your left arm.

2. **Top Leg Movement:** Slowly lift your right knee up, keeping your feet together (clamshell movement). Open your hips as far as comfortable without moving your pelvis.

3. **Hold and Breathe:** Hold the position for a few breaths, feeling the stretch in your hip and glutes.

4. **Lower and Repeat:** Slowly lower your knee back to the starting position. Repeat the movement, focusing on the gentle opening and closing of your hips.

5. **Switch Sides:** After completing the repetitions, switch to your right side and repeat the exercise.

6. **Repetition:** Perform 8-10 repetitions on each side.

### 6. *Somatic Arm Circles*

**Target Areas:** Shoulders, upper back
**Benefits:** Improves shoulder flexibility, releases tension in the upper back, and increases range of motion.

**Instructions:**

1. **Starting Position:** Stand or sit with your spine straight and arms relaxed by your sides.

2. **Raise One Arm:** Slowly lift your right arm out to the side and begin making small circles in the air with your hand. Start with clockwise circles.

3. **Expand Circles:** Gradually increase the size of the circles, exploring the full range of motion in your shoulder. Keep the movement slow and controlled.

4. **Reverse Direction:** After several circles, reverse the direction and make counterclockwise circles.

5. **Repeat on the Other Side:** Lower your right arm and repeat the sequence with your left arm.

6. **Repetition:** Perform 10-15 circles in each direction on each arm.

## 7. *Seated Forward Fold*

**Target Areas:** Hamstrings, lower back

**Benefits:** Lengthens the hamstrings, releases lower back tension, and promotes relaxation.

## Instructions:

1. **Starting Position:** Sit on the floor with your legs extended straight in front of you, feet flexed.
2. **Reach Forward:** Inhale deeply, lengthen your spine, and as you exhale, slowly reach your hands toward your feet. Keep your back as straight as possible.
3. **Gentle Stretch:** Only go as far as comfortable without forcing the stretch.

Feel the gentle lengthening in your hamstrings and lower back.

4. **Hold and Breathe:** Hold the position for several deep breaths, allowing your body to relax and deepen into the stretch with each exhale.

5. **Return to Start:** Slowly release and return to the starting position.

6. **Repetition:** Repeat 3-5 times, focusing on deepening the stretch with each repetition.

## 8. *Somatic Shoulder Bridge*

**Target Areas:** Spine, hips, hamstrings

**Benefits:** Enhances spinal flexibility, strengthens the glutes, and stretches the hip flexors.

**Instructions:**

1. **Starting Position:** Lie on your back with your knees bent and feet flat on the floor, hip-width apart. Arms should rest by your sides.

2. **Lift the Hips:** Inhale deeply, and as you exhale, slowly lift your hips toward the ceiling, creating a straight line from your shoulders to your knees.

3. **Engage and Hold:** Engage your glutes and hamstrings as you hold the bridge position for a few breaths. Keep your shoulders and neck relaxed.

4. **Lower Gently:** Slowly lower your hips back to the floor, one vertebra at a time, feeling each part of your spine make contact with the floor.

5. **Repetition:** Repeat 8-10 times, focusing on smooth and controlled movements.

### 9. *Somatic Side Bend*

**Target Areas:** Sides of the torso, shoulders, hips

**Benefits:** Increases flexibility in the sides of the torso, improves spinal mobility, and stretches the shoulders.

**Instructions:**

1. **Starting Position:** Stand or sit with your spine straight and arms relaxed by your sides.
2. **Raise One Arm:** Inhale and lift your right arm overhead, reaching toward the ceiling.
3. **Side Bend:** As you exhale, slowly bend to the left, reaching your right arm over your

head. Keep your hips stable and feel the stretch along the right side of your torso.

4. **Hold and Breathe:** Hold the side bend for a few deep breaths, deepening the stretch with each exhale.

5. **Return to Center:** Inhale as you slowly return to the starting position.

6. **Repeat on the Other Side:** Repeat the sequence on the left side, raising your left arm and bending to the right.

7. **Repetition:** Perform 3-5 side bends on each side.

## 10. *Supine Spinal Twist*

**Target Areas:** Spine, hips, shoulders
**Benefits:** Increases spinal flexibility, stretches the hips and shoulders, and promotes relaxation.

**Instructions:**

1. **Starting Position:** Lie on your back with your knees bent and feet flat on the floor.

2. **Cross One Leg:** Gently cross your right leg over your left, placing your right foot on the floor outside your left knee.

3. **Twist and Hold:** Inhale deeply, and as you exhale, slowly lower your knees to the left, allowing your right hip to lift off the floor. Extend your right arm out to the side and turn your head to the right.

4. **Breathe and Relax:** Hold the twist for several deep breaths, allowing your body to relax and deepen into the stretch.

5. **Return and Repeat:** Inhale as you slowly return to the starting position. Switch sides, crossing your left leg over your right, and repeat the twist.

6. **Repetition:** Perform 2-3 twists on each
side.

<h1 style="text-align:center">CHAPTER 5</h1>

# SOMATIC EXERCISES FOR STRENGTH

**1.** *Somatic Plank*

**Target Areas:** Core, shoulders, arms

**Benefits:** Strengthens the core, enhances shoulder stability, and improves overall body strength.

**Instructions:**

1. **Starting Position:** Begin on your hands and knees in a tabletop position. Align your wrists directly under your shoulders and your knees under your hips.

2. **Extend the Legs:** Step your feet back one at a time, straightening your legs to come into a plank position. Your body should

form a straight line from your head to your heels.

3. **Activate Your Core:** Contract your abdominal muscles to keep your hips from drooping. Visualise drawing your navel inward toward your spine.

4. **Hold the Position:** Keep your neck in a neutral position by looking slightly ahead of you. Hold the plank for 15-30 seconds, focusing on maintaining a straight line.

5. **Breathe Deeply:** Breathe evenly and deeply throughout the exercise. Avoid holding your breath.

6. **Rest and Repeat:** Lower your knees to the floor to rest, then repeat the exercise for 3-5 sets.

## 2. *Somatic Bridge Lift*

**Target Areas:** Glutes, hamstrings, lower back

**Benefits:** Strengthens the glutes and hamstrings, stabilises the lower back, and enhances hip mobility.

**Instructions:**

1. **Starting Position:** Lie on your back with your knees bent, feet flat on the floor hip-width apart, and arms resting by your sides.

2. **Engage the Core:** Inhale deeply, and as you exhale, engage your core and glutes.

3. **Lift the Hips:** Slowly lift your hips off the floor, creating a straight line from your shoulders to your knees. Engage your glutes at the peak of the motion.

4. **Hold the Position:** Hold the bridge position for 5-10 seconds, maintaining the squeeze in your glutes and a stable core.

5. **Lower and Repeat:** Lower your hips back to the floor with control, then repeat the lift for 10-15 repetitions.

6. **Repetition:** Perform 3-4 sets.

### 3. *Somatic Wall Sit*

**Target Areas:** Quads, hamstrings, glutes
**Benefits:** Strengthens the lower body, improves endurance, and enhances stability in the legs.

**Instructions:**

1. **Starting Position:** Stand with your back against a wall, feet shoulder-width apart and about 2 feet away from the wall.

2. **Lower into a Sit:** Slowly slide down the wall by bending your knees, lowering your body into a seated position. Your thighs should be parallel to the floor, and your knees directly above your ankles.

3. **Engage Your Muscles:** Hold this position by engaging your quads, hamstrings, and glutes. Keep your back pressed against the wall.

4. **Hold the Position:** Maintain the wall sit for 20-30 seconds, gradually increasing the duration as you build strength.

5. **Rest and Repeat:** Slide back up the wall to rest, then repeat the exercise for 3-4 sets.

## 4. *Somatic Chair Pose (Utkatasana)*

**Target Areas:** Quads, glutes, core

**Benefits:** Builds strength in the lower body, improves balance, and engages the core.

**Instructions:**

1. **Starting Position:** Stand with your feet together or hip-width apart, arms by your sides.

2. **Bend the Knees:** Inhale deeply, and as you exhale, bend your knees and lower your hips as if sitting back into a chair. Keep your weight in your heels.

3. **Raise the Arms:** At the same time, raise your arms overhead, keeping them in line

with your ears. Your palms should face each other.

4. **Engage the Core:** Engage your core to protect your lower back and maintain a straight spine.

5. **Hold the Pose:** Hold the chair pose for 15-30 seconds, focusing on keeping your knees aligned with your toes and your chest lifted.

6. **Return and Repeat:** Inhale as you straighten your legs to return to a standing position. Repeat for 3-5 sets.

## 5. *Somatic Push-Up*

**Target Areas:** Chest, shoulders, triceps, core
**Benefits:** Strengthens the upper body and core, improves stability, and enhances functional strength.

**Instructions:**

1. **Starting Position:** Begin in a plank position with your hands slightly wider than shoulder-width apart, feet together, and body in a straight line.

2. **Lower Your Body:** Inhale as you slowly lower your body toward the floor by bending your elbows. Keep your elbows close to your sides.

3. **Engage the Core:** Maintain a straight line from head to heels, engaging your core throughout the movement.

4. **Push Back Up:** Exhale as you push through your palms to lift your body back to the starting position.

5. **Repetition:** Perform 8-12 repetitions, focusing on smooth and controlled movements.

6. **Rest and Repeat:** Rest for a few seconds, then repeat for 3-4 sets.

### 6. *Somatic Dead Bug*

**Target Areas:** Core, lower back

**Benefits:** Strengthens the core, improves lower back stability, and enhances coordination.

### Instructions:

1. **Starting Position:** Lie on your back with your arms extended toward the ceiling and your knees bent at a 90-degree angle.

2. **Engage the Core:** Inhale deeply, and as you exhale, engage your core by pressing your lower back into the floor.

3. **Move Opposite Limbs:** Slowly lower your right arm and left leg toward the floor while keeping your lower back

pressed down. Your arm and leg should move in a controlled, simultaneous motion.

4. **Return to Start:** Inhale as you bring your arm and leg back to the starting position.

5. **Switch Sides:** Repeat the movement with your left arm and right leg.

6. **Repetition:** Perform 10-12 repetitions on each side, focusing on control and core engagement.

7. **Rest and Repeat:** Rest for a few seconds, then repeat for 3-4 sets.

### 7. *Somatic Glute Bridge March*

**Target Areas:** Glutes, hamstrings, core
**Benefits:** Strengthens the glutes and hamstrings, improves core stability, and enhances hip mobility.

**Instructions:**

1. **Starting Position:** Lie on your back with your knees bent, feet flat on the floor hip-width apart, and arms by your sides.

2. **Lift the Hips:** Inhale and lift your hips into a bridge position, creating a straight line from your shoulders to your knees.

3. **Marching Movement:** Exhale as you lift your right foot off the floor, bringing your knee toward your chest. Keep your hips stable and level.

4. **Lower the Foot:** Inhale as you lower your foot back to the floor, maintaining the bridge position.

5. **Switch Sides:** Repeat the movement with your left leg.

6. **Repetition:** Perform 8-10 repetitions on each side, focusing on stability and control.

7. **Rest and Repeat:** Lower your hips to rest, then repeat for 3-4 sets.

## 8. *Somatic Side Plank*

**Target Areas:** Obliques, shoulders, glutes

**Benefits:** Strengthens the core, particularly the obliques, improves shoulder stability, and enhances balance.

**Instructions:**

1. **Starting Position:** Begin by lying on your right side with your legs extended and stacked on top of each other. Place your right elbow directly under your shoulder.

2. **Lift the Hips:** Inhale deeply, and as you exhale, lift your hips off the floor, creating a straight line from your head to your feet. Your body should be supported by your right forearm and the side of your right foot.

3. **Engage the Core:** Tighten your abdominal muscles and keep your hips lifted.

4. **Hold the Position:** Hold the side plank for 15-30 seconds, focusing on maintaining a straight line and stable position.

5. **Lower and Switch:** Lower your hips back to the floor, then switch to your left side and repeat the exercise.

6. **Repetition:** Perform 2-3 sets on each side.

## 9. *Somatic Bird-Dog*

**Target Areas:** Core, lower back, glutes, shoulders

**Benefits:** Strengthens the core, improves balance, and enhances coordination between the upper and lower body.

**Instructions:**

1. **Starting Position:** Begin on your hands and knees in a tabletop position, with your wrists under your shoulders and your knees under your hips.

2. **Extend Opposite Limbs:** Inhale deeply, and as you exhale, extend your right arm forward and your left leg back, creating a straight line from your fingertips to your toes.

3. **Engage the Core:** Keep your core engaged and your hips level as you hold this position.

4. **Hold and Return:** Hold the position for a few breaths, then inhale as you bring your arm and leg back to the starting position.

5. **Alternate Sides:** Perform the same movement with your left arm and right leg.

6. **Repetition:** Perform 8-10 repetitions on each side, focusing on control and balance.

7. **Rest and Repeat:** Rest for a few seconds, then repeat for 3-4 sets.

## 10. *Somatic Single-Leg Stand*

**Target Areas:** Glutes, quads, core

**Benefits:** Enhances balance, strengthens the glutes and quads, and improves core stability.

**Instructions:**

1. **Starting Position:** Stand with your feet hip-width apart and your arms relaxed by your sides.

2. **Lift One Leg:** Inhale deeply, and as you exhale, lift your right leg off the floor, bending your knee slightly and bringing it toward your chest. Keep your standing leg slightly bent for stability.

3. **Engage the Core:** Tighten your abdominal muscles to maintain balance and prevent swaying.

4. **Hold the Position:** Maintain the single-leg stance for 15-30 seconds, focusing on keeping your hips level and your body steady.

5. **Lower and Switch:** Gently lower your right leg back to the floor and switch to the left leg. Repeat the same process.

6.  **Repetition:** Perform 2-3 sets on each side, gradually increasing the duration as your balance improves.

# CHAPTER 7

# SOMATIC EXERCISES FOR PAIN RELIEF

**1.** *Somatic Cat-Cow Stretch*

**Target Areas:** Spine, lower back, shoulders
**Benefits:** Relieves lower back pain, improves spinal flexibility, and releases tension in the shoulders.

**Instructions:**

1. **Starting Position:** Begin on your hands and knees in a tabletop position. Position your wrists directly beneath your shoulders and your knees directly under your hips.

2. **Cat Pose (Flexion):** Inhale deeply, and as you exhale, round your back toward the ceiling, tucking your chin to your chest. This stretches the spine and relieves lower back tension.

3. **Cow Pose (Extension):** Inhale as you lower your belly toward the floor, arching your back and lifting your head and tailbone. This opens the chest and stretches the lower back.

4. **Flow Between Poses:** Continue to move between Cat and Cow poses with each breath, allowing the spine to flex and extend.

5. **Repetition:** Perform 10-12 cycles, focusing on the gentle release of tension with each movement.

## 2. *Somatic Child's Pose*

**Target Areas:** Lower back, hips, shoulders
**Benefits:** Relieves tension in the lower back and hips, and gently stretches the shoulders.

**Instructions:**

1. **Starting Position:** Kneel on the floor with your knees wide apart and toes touching. Sit back on your heels.
2. **Extend the Arms:** Inhale deeply, and as you exhale, extend your arms forward on the floor, lowering your torso between your thighs.

3. **Relax and Breathe:** Rest your forehead on the floor and allow your arms to stretch forward. Breathe deeply, letting go of tension in your lower back and shoulders.

4. **Hold the Pose:** Stay in this position for 30-60 seconds, feeling the gentle stretch and release in your back and hips.

5. **Return and Repeat:** Slowly come back to the starting position. Repeat as needed for comfort.

### 3. *Somatic Supine Twist*

**Target Areas:** Spine, lower back, hips

**Benefits:** Relieves lower back pain, stretches the spine, and releases tension in the hips.

**Instructions:**

1. **Starting Position:** Lie on your back with your knees bent and feet flat on the floor.

2. **Cross the Legs:** Gently cross your right leg over your left, placing your right foot outside your left knee.

3. **Twist the Spine:** Inhale deeply, and as you exhale, let your knees fall to the left side of your body. Extend your right arm out to the side and turn your head to the right.

4. **Hold and Breathe:** Hold this position for 30-60 seconds, feeling the stretch in your spine and hips.

5. **Return and Switch:** Slowly return to the starting position and repeat on the other side.

### 4. *Somatic Seated Forward Fold*

**Target Areas:** Hamstrings, lower back

**Benefits:** Relieves lower back pain, stretches the hamstrings, and promotes relaxation.

## Instructions:

1. **Starting Position:** Sit on the floor with your legs extended straight in front of you, feet flexed.

2. **Reach Forward:** Inhale deeply, lengthening your spine, and as you exhale, slowly reach your hands toward your feet, keeping your back straight.

3. **Gently Fold:** Only go as far as comfortable without forcing the stretch. Feel the gentle lengthening in your hamstrings and lower back.

4. **Hold and Breathe:** Stay in this position for 30-60 seconds, allowing your body to relax and release tension.

5. **Return to Start:** Slowly come back up to a seated position. Repeat if desired.

## 5. *Somatic Side-Lying Leg Stretch*

**Target Areas:** Hips, lower back

**Benefits:** Relieves hip and lower back tension, and improves flexibility in the hips.

**Instructions:**

1. **Starting Position:** Lie on your left side with your legs extended and stacked on top of each other. Rest your head on your left arm.

2. **Bend the Top Knee:** Bend your right knee and bring it toward your chest. Grasp your right ankle with your right hand.

3. **Gently Stretch:** Gently pull your right ankle toward your glutes, feeling the stretch in your hip and lower back.

4. **Hold and Breathe:** Maintain this stretch for 30-60 seconds, focusing on the release of tension.

5. **Switch Sides:** Slowly release and switch to the other side, repeating the stretch with your left knee.

## 6. *Somatic Upper Back Stretch*

**Target Areas:** Upper back, shoulders

**Benefits:** Relieves tension in the upper back and shoulders, and improves posture.

**Instructions:**

1. **Starting Position:** Sit or stand with your spine straight and your arms extended in front of you.

2. **Cross the Arms:** Bring your arms out in front of you and cross your right arm over your left.

3. **Hug and Stretch:** Wrap your arms around each other, bringing your palms to touch if possible. Press your hands away from you and round your upper back.

4. **Hold and Breathe:** Hold the stretch for 30-60 seconds, feeling the release in your upper back and shoulders.

5. **Switch Arms:** Release and switch to cross your left arm over your right, repeating the stretch.

### 7. *Somatic Reclining Hand-to-Big-Toe Pose*

**Target Areas:** Hamstrings, lower back

**Benefits:** Stretches the hamstrings, releases lower back tension, and improves flexibility.

**Instructions:**

1. **Starting Position:** Lie on your back with your right leg extended straight and left knee bent.

2. **Raise the Leg:** Inhale deeply, and as you exhale, use a strap or your hand to lift your right leg toward the ceiling, keeping it straight.

3. **Gently Stretch:** Hold the stretch for 30-60 seconds, feeling the lengthening in your hamstrings and lower back.

4. **Switch Sides:** Slowly lower your right leg and repeat the stretch with your left leg.

## 8. *Somatic Gentle Neck Stretch*

**Target Areas:** Neck, shoulders

**Benefits:** Relieves neck and shoulder tension, and improves flexibility in the neck.

**Instructions:**

1. **Starting Position:** Sit or stand with your spine straight and shoulders relaxed.
2. **Tilt the Head:** Slowly tilt your right ear toward your right shoulder, feeling a gentle stretch on the left side of your neck.
3. **Use the Hand:** For a deeper stretch, gently press your left temple with your left hand. Avoid straining.
4. **Hold and Breathe:** Hold this position for 30-60 seconds, allowing the stretch to deepen with each exhale.
5. **Switch Sides:** Slowly return to the starting position and repeat on the left side.

## 9. *Somatic Reclining Spinal Twist*

**Target Areas:** Spine, hips

**Benefits:** Relieves lower back pain, stretches the spine, and improves flexibility in the hips.

**Instructions:**

1. **Starting Position:** Lie on your back with your knees bent and feet flat on the floor.

2. **Cross the Legs:** Gently cross your right knee over your left, placing your right foot outside your left knee.

3. **Twist the Spine:** Inhale deeply, and as you exhale, let your knees fall to the left while extending your right arm out to the side and turning your head to the right.

4. **Hold and Breathe:** Hold the twist for 30-60 seconds, feeling the stretch in your spine and hips.

5. **Return and Switch:** Return to the starting position and repeat on the other side.

## 10. *Somatic Hip Flexor Stretch*

**Target Areas:** Hip flexors, quads

**Benefits:** Relieves tension in the hip flexors, reduces lower back pain, and improves hip mobility.

**Instructions:**

1. **Starting Position:** Kneel on your right knee with your left foot in front, forming a 90-degree angle at both knees.

2. **Push Hips Forward:** Inhale deeply, and as you exhale, gently push your hips

forward, feeling a stretch in your right hip flexor.

3. **Engage Your Core:** Keep your torso upright and your core engaged to support your lower back.

4. **Hold and Breathe:** Hold the stretch for 30-60 seconds, focusing on relaxing into the stretch.

5. **Switch Sides:** Gently release the stretch and switch to kneel on your left knee, repeating the stretch with your right leg in front.

# CHAPTER 8

# SOMATIC FOR ENHANCING BALANCE AND COORDINATION

1. *Somatic Tree Pose*

**Target Areas:** Balance, core, legs

**Benefits:** Improves balance, strengthens the core, and enhances coordination between the upper and lower body.

**Instructions:**

1. **Starting Position:** Stand with your feet hip-width apart and your arms relaxed by your sides.

2. **Shift Weight:** Slowly shift your weight onto your left foot. Bend your right knee and place your right foot on your left inner thigh or calf (avoid the knee).

3. **Find Your Balance:** Engage your core and keep your gaze fixed on a point ahead to maintain balance.

4. **Raise the Arms:** Inhale as you raise your arms overhead, bringing your palms together or keeping them apart.

5. **Hold the Pose:** Maintain the pose for 20-30 seconds, focusing on your balance and breathing steadily.

6. **Switch Sides:** Lower your right foot and repeat on the left side.

## 2. *Somatic Warrior III*

**Target Areas:** Core, legs, balance

**Benefits:** Strengthens the core and legs, and improves balance and coordination.

**Instructions:**

1. **Starting Position:** Stand with your feet hip-width apart and your arms by your sides.

2. **Prepare to Lift:** Shift your weight onto your left foot and engage your core.

3. **Lift and Extend:** Inhale as you lift your right leg behind you, keeping it straight and parallel to the floorReach your arms forward, keeping them parallel to the floor.

4. **Maintain Balance:** Hold this position for 15-30 seconds, focusing on keeping your torso and leg in a straight line.

5. **Return and Switch:** Lower your leg and arms to return to the starting position. Repeat on the other side.

### 3. *Somatic Single-Leg Deadlift*

**Target Areas:** Core, hamstrings, balance

**Benefits:** Improves balance, strengthens the hamstrings, and enhances core stability.

**Instructions:**

1. **Starting Position:** Stand with your feet hip-width apart and your hands resting on your hips.

2. **Shift Weight:** Shift your weight onto your left foot and engage your core.

3. **Extend the Leg:** Inhale as you hinge forward from your hips, extending your right leg behind you and reaching your arms toward the floor.

4. **Hold the Position:** Keep your back flat and your core engaged. Hold for 10-20 seconds, focusing on balance.

5. **Return and Switch:** Return to the starting position and repeat with the other leg.

### 4. *Somatic Standing March*

**Target Areas:** Core, legs, coordination
**Benefits:** Enhances coordination, improves core stability, and strengthens the legs.

**Instructions:**

1. **Starting Position:** Stand with your feet hip-width apart and your arms by your sides.

2. **Begin Marching:** Lift your right knee toward your chest while simultaneously swinging your left arm forward.

3. **Alternate Legs:** Lower your right leg and arm, then lift your left knee and swing your right arm forward.

4. **Maintain Rhythm:** Continue marching in place, focusing on coordinating the movement of your arms and legs.

5. **Duration:** March for 1-2 minutes, maintaining a steady rhythm.

### 5. *Somatic Heel-to-Toe Walk*

**Target Areas:** Balance, coordination

**Benefits:** Improves balance and coordination by

challenging your stability with a focused walking exercise.

**Instructions:**

1. **Starting Position:** Stand with your feet together and arms by your sides.
2. **Start Walking:** Take a step forward with your right foot, placing the heel directly in front of the toes of your left foot.
3. **Continue Walking:** Follow with your left foot, placing the heel directly in front of the toes of your right foot.
4. **Focus on Balance:** Continue walking in this manner, maintaining a straight line and focusing on balance.
5. **Distance:** Walk in a straight line for about 10-15 steps, then turn and walk back.

**6. Somatic Balance on Toes**

**Target Areas:** Balance, calves, core

**Benefits:** Strengthens the calves, enhances balance, and improves core stability.

**Instructions:**

1. **Starting Position:** Stand with your feet hip-width apart and your arms by your sides.
2. **Rise onto Toes:** Slowly lift your heels off the floor, coming up onto the balls of your feet.
3. **Maintain Balance:** Hold this position for 10-20 seconds, keeping your core engaged and your gaze fixed ahead.
4. **Lower and Repeat:** Lower your heels back to the floor and repeat for 2-3 sets.

### 7. *Somatic Side Leg Raises*

**Target Areas:** Hips, core, balance

**Benefits:** Strengthens the hip muscles, improves balance, and enhances core stability.

**Instructions:**

1. **Starting Position:** Stand with your feet together and your hands resting on your hips or holding onto a wall for support.
2. **Lift One Leg:** Shift your weight onto your left leg and slowly lift your right leg out to the side, keeping it straight.
3. **Hold and Lower:** Hold the leg in the lifted position for 5-10 seconds, then lower it back to the starting position.
4. **Switch Sides:** Repeat with the left leg. Perform 10-15 repetitions on each side.

### 8. *Somatic Tadasana (Mountain Pose)*

**Target Areas:** Core, legs, posture

**Benefits:** Improves posture, enhances balance, and strengthens the core and legs.

**Instructions:**

1. **Starting Position:** Stand with your feet together or hip-width apart, arms by your sides.
2. **Engage the Core:** Inhale deeply, engaging your core muscles and lifting your chest.
3. **Ground the Feet:** Press evenly through the soles of your feet and distribute your weight evenly.
4. **Maintain the Pose:** Hold this position for 20-30 seconds, focusing on your posture and balance.
5. **Relax and Repeat:** Release the pose and repeat if desired.

## 9. *Somatic Seated Balance*

**Target Areas:** Core, balance

**Benefits:** Enhances balance and core stability while seated, which is ideal for beginners.

**Instructions:**

1. **Starting Position:** Sit on a chair with your feet flat on the floor and your hands resting on your thighs.
2. **Lift One Foot:** Slowly lift your right foot off the floor, extending your leg slightly.
3. **Hold and Balance:** Hold the leg in the lifted position for 10-20 seconds, engaging your core to maintain balance.

4. **Switch Feet:** Lower your right foot and repeat with your left foot.

5. **Repetition:** Perform 5-10 repetitions on each side, focusing on control and stability.

**10.** *Somatic Alternating Arm and Leg Lift*

**Target Areas:** Core, balance, coordination

**Benefits:** Strengthens the core, improves coordination between the upper and lower body, and enhances balance.

**Instructions:**

1. **Starting Position:** Begin on your hands and knees in a tabletop position.

2. **Extend Opposite Limbs:** Inhale as you extend your right arm forward and your

left leg back, keeping both straight and parallel to the floor.

3. **Hold and Engage:** Hold this position for 5-10 seconds, engaging your core to maintain stability.

4. **Return and Switch:** Lower your arm and leg back to the starting position and repeat with your left arm and right leg.

5. **Repetition:** Perform 8-10 repetitions on each side, focusing on smooth and controlled movements.

# CHAPTER 8

# SOMATIC EXERCISES FOR STRESS RELIEF

**1.** *Somatic Tree Pose*

**Target Areas:** Balance, core, legs

**Benefits:** Improves balance, strengthens the core, and enhances coordination between the upper and lower body.

**Instructions:**

1. **Starting Position:** Stand with your feet hip-width apart and your arms relaxed by your sides.

2. **Shift Weight:** Slowly shift your weight onto your left foot. Bend your right knee and position your right foot on your left inner thigh or calf, avoiding the knee.

3. **Find Your Balance:** Engage your core and keep your gaze fixed on a point ahead to maintain balance.

4. **Raise the Arms:** Inhale as you raise your arms overhead, bringing your palms together or keeping them apart.

5. **Hold the Pose:** Maintain the pose for 20-30 seconds, focusing on your balance and breathing steadily.

6. **Switch Sides:** Lower your right foot and repeat on the left side.

## 2. *Somatic Warrior III*

**Target Areas:** Core, legs, balance

**Benefits:** Strengthens the core and legs, and improves balance and coordination.

**Instructions:**

1. **Starting Position:** Stand with your feet hip-width apart and your arms by your sides.

2. **Prepare to Lift:** Shift your weight onto your left foot and engage your core.

3. **Lift and Extend:** Inhale as you lift your right leg behind you, keeping it straight and parallel to the floor.Stretch your arms forward, maintaining them parallel to the floor.

4. **Maintain Balance:** Hold this position for 15-30 seconds, focusing on keeping your torso and leg in a straight line.

5. **Return and Switch:** Lower your leg and arms to return to the starting position. Repeat on the other side.

### 3. *Somatic Single-Leg Deadlift*

**Target Areas:** Core, hamstrings, balance

**Benefits:** Improves balance, strengthens the hamstrings, and enhances core stability.

**Instructions:**

1. **Starting Position:** Stand with your feet hip-width apart and your hands resting on your hips.

2. **Shift Weight:** Shift your weight onto your left foot and engage your core.

3. **Extend the Leg:** Inhale as you hinge forward from your hips, extending your right leg behind you and reaching your arms toward the floor.

4. **Hold the Position:** Keep your back flat and your core engaged. Hold for 10-20 seconds, focusing on balance.

5. **Return and Switch:** Return to the starting position and repeat with the other leg.

## 4. *Somatic Standing March*

**Target Areas:** Core, legs, coordination

**Benefits:** Enhances coordination, improves core stability, and strengthens the legs.

**Instructions:**

1. **Starting Position:** Stand with your feet hip-width apart and your arms by your sides.

2. **Begin Marching:** Lift your right knee toward your chest while simultaneously swinging your left arm forward.

3. **Alternate Legs:** Lower your right leg and arm, then lift your left knee and swing your right arm forward.

4. **Maintain Rhythm:** Continue marching in place, focusing on coordinating the movement of your arms and legs.

5. **Duration:** March for 1-2 minutes, maintaining a steady rhythm.

### 5. *Somatic Heel-to-Toe Walk*

**Target Areas:** Balance, coordination

**Benefits:** Improves balance and coordination by

challenging your stability with a focused walking exercise.

**Instructions:**

1. **Starting Position:** Stand with your feet together and arms by your sides.
2. **Start Walking:** Take a step forward with your right foot, placing the heel directly in front of the toes of your left foot.
3. **Continue Walking:** Follow with your left foot, placing the heel directly in front of the toes of your right foot.
4. **Focus on Balance:** Continue walking in this manner, maintaining a straight line and focusing on balance.
5. **Distance:** Walk in a straight line for about 10-15 steps, then turn and walk back.

### 6. *Somatic Balance on Toes*

**Target Areas:** Balance, calves, core

**Benefits:** Strengthens the calves, enhances balance, and improves core stability.

**Instructions:**

1. **Starting Position:** Stand with your feet hip-width apart and your arms by your sides.

2. **Rise onto Toes:** Slowly lift your heels off the floor, coming up onto the balls of your feet.

3. **Maintain Balance:** Hold this position for 10-20 seconds, keeping your core engaged and your gaze fixed ahead.

4. **Lower and Repeat:** Lower your heels back to the floor and repeat for 2-3 sets.

### 7. *Somatic Side Leg Raises*

**Target Areas:** Hips, core, balance

**Benefits:** Strengthens the hip muscles, improves balance, and enhances core stability.

**Instructions:**

1. **Starting Position:** Stand with your feet together and your hands resting on your hips or holding onto a wall for support.
2. **Lift One Leg:** Shift your weight onto your left leg and slowly lift your right leg out to the side, keeping it straight.
3. **Hold and Lower:** Hold the leg in the lifted position for 5-10 seconds, then lower it back to the starting position.
4. **Switch Sides:** Repeat with the left leg. Perform 10-15 repetitions on each side.

### 8. *Somatic Tadasana (Mountain Pose)*

**Target Areas:** Core, legs, posture

**Benefits:** Improves posture, enhances balance, and strengthens the core and legs.

**Instructions:**

1. **Starting Position:** Stand with your feet together or hip-width apart, arms by your sides.
2. **Engage the Core:** Inhale deeply, engaging your core muscles and lifting your chest.
3. **Ground the Feet:** Press evenly through the soles of your feet and distribute your weight evenly.
4. **Maintain the Pose:** Hold this position for 20-30 seconds, focusing on your posture and balance.
5. **Relax and Repeat:** Release the pose and repeat if desired.

## 9. *Somatic Seated Balance*

**Target Areas:** Core, balance

**Benefits:** Enhances balance and core stability while seated, which is ideal for beginners.

**Instructions:**

1. **Starting Position:** Sit on a chair with your feet flat on the floor and your hands resting on your thighs.
2. **Lift One Foot:** Slowly lift your right foot off the floor, extending your leg slightly.
3. **Hold and Balance:** Hold the leg in the lifted position for 10-20 seconds, engaging your core to maintain balance.
4. **Switch Feet:** Lower your right foot and repeat with your left foot.

5. **Repetition:** Perform 5-10 repetitions on each side, focusing on control and stability.

## 10. *Somatic Alternating Arm and Leg Lift*

**Target Areas:** Core, balance, coordination

**Benefits:** Strengthens the core, improves coordination between the upper and lower body, and enhances balance.

**Instructions:**

1. **Starting Position:** Begin on your hands and knees in a tabletop position.
2. **Extend Opposite Limbs:** Inhale as you extend your right arm forward and your left leg back, keeping both straight and parallel to the floor.

3. **Hold and Engage:** Hold this position for 5-10 seconds, engaging your core to maintain stability.

4. **Return and Switch:** Lower your arm and leg back to the starting position and repeat with your left arm and right leg.

5. **Repetition:** Perform 8-10 repetitions on each side, focusing on smooth and controlled movements.

1. **Starting Position:** Stand with your feet hip-width apart and your arms relaxed by your sides.

2. **Fold Forward:** Inhale deeply, and as you exhale, slowly fold forward at your hips, letting your arms dangle toward the floor.

3. **Relax the Neck:** Allow your head and neck to relax completely, feeling the

gentle stretch in your lower back and hamstrings.

4. **Hold and Breathe:** Stay in this position for 30-60 seconds, breathing deeply and releasing tension.

5. **Return:** Slowly roll up to a standing position, one vertebra at a time.

# SECTION III

# CHAPTER 10

# INTEGRATING SOMATIC EXERCISES INTO YOUR DAILY ROUTINE

Welcome to the third section of your somatic journey, where we focus on integrating these transformative exercises into your daily life. In this section, we will guide you through a structured 4-week workout plan designed to help you make somatic exercises an effortless part of your routine. Whether you're new to somatics or looking to deepen your practice, this plan will provide the support you need to achieve your goals.

## The 4-Week Workout Plan

Our 4-week workout plan is crafted to encompass a variety of somatic poses, categorised to address different aspects of well-being. The plan includes:

1. Somatic Exercises for Flexibility

2. Somatic Exercises for Strength

3. Somatic Exercises for Pain Relief

4. Enhancing Balance and Coordination

5. Somatic Exercises for Stress Relief

Each category targets specific areas of physical and mental health, ensuring a comprehensive approach to your practice.

**Daily Structure:** Each day features two specific exercises—one for the morning and one for the evening. This balanced approach helps you start your day with energy and end it with relaxation. By incorporating a diverse range of somatic poses, you'll experience improvements in flexibility, strength, pain relief, balance, and stress management.

**Example of Daily Routine:**

- **Morning Exercise:** Focuses on energizing and preparing your body for the day.

- **Evening Exercise:** Aims to relax and restore, helping you unwind and de-stress before bed.

**Categories and Benefits:**

1. **Somatic Exercises for Flexibility:** These exercises enhance your body's range of motion and reduce stiffness, helping you move with greater ease and comfort.

2. **Somatic Exercises for Strength:** Targeted poses to build and maintain muscle strength, contributing to overall physical stability and endurance.

3. **Somatic Exercises for Pain Relief:** Gentle movements designed to alleviate chronic pain and improve your body's natural healing processes.

4. **Enhancing Balance and Coordination:** Exercises that improve your body's

balance and coordination, reducing the risk of falls and enhancing overall functional movement.

5. **Somatic Exercises for Stress Relief:** Poses that promote relaxation and mental clarity, helping you manage stress and find tranquility in your daily life.

## RECORDING JOURNAL AND TRACKER

To ensure that you stay motivated and track your progress effectively, we have included a **Recording Journal** and a **Tracker**:

- **Recording Journal:** Use this journal to document your daily practice, noting the exercises performed, your feelings before and after each session, and any observations or improvements. This tool will help you reflect on your journey and adjust your routine as needed.

- **Tracker:** The tracker allows you to visually monitor your progress over the 4 weeks. Mark off each exercise completed and review your achievements regularly to stay on track and celebrate your progress.

By following this 4-week workout plan, you'll not only integrate somatic exercises into your daily routine but also experience the many benefits of a holistic and mindful approach to movement. Embrace this journey with an open mind, and allow these exercises to enrich your life, enhance your well-being, and support your personal growth.

Get ready to start your daily routine and experience the transformative power of somatic exercises. Your path to improved flexibility, strength, pain relief, balance, and stress relief begins here.

# CHAPTER 11

# 4-Week Workout Plan: Day 1 to Day 30

This 30-day plan provides a structured approach to integrating somatic exercises into your daily routine. Each day includes two exercises—one for the morning and one for the evening—to help you build flexibility, strength, balance, and stress relief while addressing pain.

# WEEK 1

## Day 1

- **Morning: Seated Forward Bend** *(Somatic Exercises for Flexibility)*
    - **Description:** Sit with your legs extended in front of you. Inhale deeply, and as you exhale, gently fold forward, reaching towards your feet.
    - **Duration:** Hold for 30 seconds to 1 minute.
- **Evening: Seated Shoulder Shrugs** *(Somatic Exercises for Stress Relief)*
    - **Description:** Lift your shoulders towards your ears, then roll them back and down.

○ **Duration:** Perform 10-15 shoulder shrugs.

**Day 2**

- **Morning: Seated Arm Circles** *(Somatic Exercises for Strength)*
  ○ **Description:** Extend your arms out to the sides at shoulder height and make small circles in the air.
  ○ **Duration:** 1 minute in each direction.
- **Evening: Seated Gentle Twist** *(Somatic Exercises for Pain Relief)*
  ○ **Description:** Sit with your legs crossed. Place your right hand on your left knee and twist your torso gently to the left. Hold, then switch sides.

    ○ **Duration:** Hold each side for 30 seconds.

## Day 3

- **Morning: Seated Side Stretch** *(Somatic Exercises for Flexibility)*
  - **Description:** Sit with your legs extended and reach your right arm over your head while leaning to the left. Hold, then switch sides.
  - **Duration:** Hold each side for 30 seconds.
- **Evening: Seated Foot Taps** *(Enhancing Balance and Coordination)*
  - **Description:** Sit with your feet flat on the floor. Alternate tapping your toes on the floor while keeping your heels grounded.
  - **Duration:** Perform for 1 minute.

**Day 4**

- **Morning: Seated Spine Twist** *(Somatic Exercises for Flexibility)*
    - **Description:** Sit with your legs crossed. Twist your torso to the right and hold with your left hand on your right knee. Switch sides.
    - **Duration:** Hold each side for 30 seconds.
- **Evening: Seated Warrior Pose** *(Somatic Exercises for Strength)*
    - **Description:** Sit with your right foot flat on the floor and extend your left leg out straight. Raise your arms to shoulder height and hold.
    - **Duration:** Hold for 30 seconds to 1 minute on each side.

**Day 5**

- **Morning: Seated Neck Rolls** *(Somatic Exercises for Stress Relief)*
  - **Description:** Sit with your spine straight. Slowly roll your head in a circular motion, first clockwise, then counterclockwise.
  - **Duration:** 30 seconds in each direction.
- **Evening: Seated Leg Extensions** *(Somatic Exercises for Strength)*
  - **Description:** Sit with your back straight and extend one leg out straight, holding for a moment, then switch legs.
  - **Duration:** Hold each leg for 20-30 seconds.

**Day 6**

- **Morning: Seated Cat-Cow Stretch** *(Somatic Exercises for Flexibility)*
  - **Description:** Sit with your hands on your knees. Arch your back and look up (Cow Pose), then round your back and tuck your chin (Cat Pose).
  - **Duration:** Alternate between poses for 1 minute.
- **Evening: Seated Butterfly Stretch** *(Somatic Exercises for Pain Relief)*
  - **Description:** Sit with your feet together and knees out to the sides. Gently press your knees down while leaning forward.
  - **Duration:** Hold for 30-60 seconds.

**Day 7**

- **Morning: Seated March** *(Enhancing Balance and Coordination)*
  - **Description:** Sit with your back straight and lift one knee towards your chest, alternating legs.
  - **Duration:** Perform for 1 minute.
- **Evening: Seated Chest Opener** *(Somatic Exercises for Stress Relief)*
  - **Description:** Sit with your hands clasped behind your back and gently lift your arms while opening your chest.
  - **Duration:** Hold for 30 seconds.

# WEEK 2

**Day 8**

- **Morning: Seated Side Bend** *(Somatic Exercises for Flexibility)*
  - **Description:** Sit with your legs extended. Reach your left arm over your head and lean to the right, then switch sides.
  - **Duration:** Hold each side for 30-45 seconds.
- **Evening: Seated Shoulder Shrugs** *(Somatic Exercises for Stress Relief)*
  - **Description:** Lift and lower your shoulders, rolling them backward.
  - **Duration:** Perform 15-20 shoulder shrugs.

**Day 9**

- **Morning: Seated Arm Circles** *(Somatic Exercises for Strength)*
    - **Description:** Extend your arms out to the sides and make small circles, reversing direction after 1 minute.
    - **Duration:** 1 minute in each direction.
- **Evening: Seated Gentle Twist** *(Somatic Exercises for Pain Relief)*
    - **Description:** Twist your torso gently while sitting, switching sides after 30 seconds.
    - **Duration:** Hold each side for 30-45 seconds.

**Day 10**

- **Morning: Seated Forward Bend** *(Somatic Exercises for Flexibility)*
  - ○ **Description:** Fold forward from a seated position, reaching towards your feet.
  - ○ **Duration:** Hold for 45 seconds to 1 minute.
- **Evening: Seated Foot Taps** *(Enhancing Balance and Coordination)*
  - ○ **Description:** Alternate tapping your toes on the floor while keeping heels grounded.
  - ○ **Duration:** Perform for 1-2 minutes.

**Day 11**

- **Morning: Seated Spine Twist** *(Somatic Exercises for Flexibility)* o **Description:** Twist your torso gently, holding each side.

o **Duration:** Hold each side for 30-45 seconds.

- **Evening: Seated Warrior Pose** *(Somatic Exercises for Strength)*

    o **Description:** Extend one leg out straight with arms raised, holding the pose.

    o **Duration:** Hold for 45 seconds to 1 minute on each side.

## Day 12

- **Morning: Seated Neck Rolls** *(Somatic Exercises for Stress Relief)*

    o **Description:** Roll your head in a circular motion.

- ○ **Duration:** 45 seconds in each direction.
- **Evening: Seated Leg Extensions** *(Somatic Exercises for Strength)*
  - ○ **Description:** Extend one leg out straight, then switch legs.
  - ○ **Duration:** Hold each leg for 30 seconds.

**Day 13**

- **Morning: Seated Cat-Cow Stretch** *(Somatic Exercises for Flexibility)*
  - ○ **Description:** Alternate between arching and rounding your back.
  - ○ **Duration:** Continue for 1-2 minutes.
- **Evening: Seated Butterfly Stretch** *(Somatic Exercises for Pain Relief)*

- Description: Press your knees down while leaning forward.
  - Duration: Hold for 45-60 seconds.

**Day 14**

- **Morning: Seated March** *(Enhancing Balance and Coordination)*
  - **Description:** Lift one knee towards your chest, alternating legs.
  - **Duration:** Perform for 1-2 minutes.
- **Evening: Seated Chest Opener** *(Somatic Exercises for Stress Relief)*
  - **Description:** Open your chest by lifting your clasped hands behind your back.
  - **Duration:** Hold for 45 seconds.

## WEEK 3

**Day 15**

- **Morning: Seated Side Stretch** *(Somatic Exercises for Flexibility)*
  - **Description:** Sit with your legs extended. Reach your right arm overhead and lean to the left, then switch sides.
  - **Duration:** Hold each side for 45 seconds.
- **Evening: Seated Neck Rolls** *(Somatic Exercises for Stress Relief)*
  - **Description:** Roll your head gently in circular motions.
  - **Duration:** 1 minute in each direction.

**Day 16**

- **Morning: Seated Arm Circles** *(Somatic Exercises for Strength)*
  - **Description:** Make small circles with your arms extended out to the sides.
  - **Duration:** 1 minute in each direction.
- **Evening: Seated Gentle Twist** *(Somatic Exercises for Pain Relief)*
  - **Description:** Twist your torso to each side, holding the stretch.
  - **Duration:** Hold each side for 45 seconds.

**Day 17**

- **Morning: Seated Forward Bend** *(Somatic Exercises for Flexibility)*

- o **Description:** Reach forward towards your feet while seated.
  - o **Duration:** Hold for 1 minute.
- **Evening: Seated Foot Taps** *(Enhancing Balance and Coordination)*
  - o **Description:** Alternate tapping your toes on the floor while keeping heels grounded.
  - o **Duration:** Perform for 1-2 minutes.

**Day 18**

- **Morning: Seated Spine Twist** *(Somatic Exercises for Flexibility)*
  - o **Description:** Twist your torso gently, holding each side.
  - o **Duration:** Hold each side for 45 seconds.

- **Evening: Seated Warrior Pose** *(Somatic Exercises for Strength)*
  - **Description:** Extend one leg out straight with arms raised, holding the pose.
  - **Duration:** Hold for 1 minute on each side.

**Day 19**

- **Morning: Seated Neck Rolls** *(Somatic Exercises for Stress Relief)*
  - **Description:** Roll your head gently in circular motions.
  - **Duration:** 1 minute in each direction.
- **Evening: Seated Leg Extensions** *(Somatic Exercises for Strength)*

o **Description:** Extend one leg out straight, then switch legs.

o **Duration:** Hold each leg for 30 seconds.

**Day 20**

- **Morning: Seated Cat-Cow Stretch** *(Somatic Exercises for Flexibility)*

  o **Description:** Alternate between arching and rounding your back.

  o **Duration:** Continue for 1-2 minutes.

- **Evening: Seated Butterfly Stretch** *(Somatic Exercises for Pain Relief)*

  o **Description:** Press your knees down while leaning forward.

  o **Duration:** Hold for 1 minute.

**Day 21**

- **Morning: Seated March** *(Enhancing Balance and Coordination)*
    - o **Description:** Lift one knee towards your chest, alternating legs.
    - o **Duration:** Perform for 1-2 minutes.
- **Evening: Seated Chest Opener** *(Somatic Exercises for Stress Relief)*
    - o **Description:** Open your chest by lifting your clasped hands behind your back.
    - o **Duration:** Hold for 1 minute.

# WEEK 4

**Day 22**

- **Morning: Seated Side Stretch** *(Somatic Exercises for Flexibility)*
    - **Description:** Sit with your legs extended. Reach your left arm overhead and lean to the right, then switch sides.
    - **Duration:** Hold each side for 45 seconds.
- **Evening: Seated Neck Rolls** *(Somatic Exercises for Stress Relief)*
    - **Description:** Roll your head gently in circular motions.
    - **Duration:** 1 minute in each direction.

**Day 23**

- **Morning: Seated Arm Circles** *(Somatic Exercises for Strength)*
    - **Description:** Make small circles with your arms extended out to the sides.
    - **Duration:** 1 minute in each direction.
- **Evening: Seated Gentle Twist** *(Somatic Exercises for Pain Relief)*
    - **Description:** Twist your torso to each side, holding the stretch.
    - **Duration:** Hold each side for 45 seconds.

**Day 24**

- **Morning: Seated Forward Bend** *(Somatic Exercises for Flexibility)*

- **Description:** Reach forward towards your feet while seated.
  - **Duration:** Hold for 1 minute.
- **Evening: Seated Foot Taps** *(Enhancing Balance and Coordination)*
  - **Description:** Alternate tapping your toes on the floor while keeping heels grounded.
  - **Duration:** Perform for 1-2 minutes.

## Day 25

- **Morning: Seated Spine Twist** *(Somatic Exercises for Flexibility)*
  - **Description:** Twist your torso gently, holding each side.
  - **Duration:** Hold each side for 1 minute.

- **Evening: Seated Warrior Pose** *(Somatic Exercises for Strength)*
  - **Description:** Extend one leg out straight with arms raised, holding the pose.
  - **Duration:** Hold for 1 minute on each side.

**Day 26**

- **Morning: Seated Neck Rolls** *(Somatic Exercises for Stress Relief)*
  - **Description:** Roll your head gently in circular motions.
  - **Duration:** 1 minute in each direction.
- **Evening: Seated Leg Extensions** *(Somatic Exercises for Strength)*

o **Description:** Extend one leg out straight, then switch legs.

o **Duration:** Hold each leg for 30 seconds.

**Day 27**

- **Morning: Seated Cat-Cow Stretch** *(Somatic Exercises for Flexibility)*

    o **Description:** Alternate between arching and rounding your back.

    o **Duration:** Continue for 1-2 minutes.

- **Evening: Seated Butterfly Stretch** *(Somatic Exercises for Pain Relief)*

    o **Description:** Press your knees down while leaning forward.

    o **Duration:** Hold for 1 minute.

**Day 28**

- **Morning: Seated March** *(Enhancing Balance and Coordination)*
  - ○ **Description:** Lift one knee towards your chest, alternating legs.
  - ○ **Duration:** Perform for 1-2 minutes.
- **Evening: Seated Chest Opener** *(Somatic Exercises for Stress Relief)*
  - ○ **Description:** Open your chest by lifting your clasped hands behind your back.
  - ○ **Duration:** Hold for 1 minute.

**Day 29**

- **Morning: Seated Side Stretch** *(Somatic Exercises for Flexibility)*
  - ○ **Description:** Sit with your legs extended. Reach your right arm

overhead and lean to the left, then switch sides.

- o **Duration:** Hold each side for 1 minute.

- **Evening: Seated Neck Rolls** *(Somatic Exercises for Stress Relief)*

  - o **Description:** Roll your head gently in circular motions.
  - o **Duration:** 1 minute in each direction.

**Day 30**

- **Morning: Seated Arm Circles** *(Somatic Exercises for Strength)*

  - o **Description:** Make small circles with your arms extended out to the sides.
  - o **Duration:** 1 minute in each direction.

- **Evening: Seated Gentle Twist** *(Somatic Exercises for Pain Relief)*
    - **Description:** Twist your torso to each side, holding the stretch.
    - **Duration:** Hold each side for 1 minute.

# CHAPTER 12

# TRACKER AND JOURNAL

| DAYS | EXERCISES | CHECK |
|------|-----------|-------|
|  |  |  |
|  |  |  |
|  |  |  |
|  |  |  |
|  |  |  |
|  |  |  |
|  |  |  |
|  |  |  |
|  |  |  |
|  |  |  |
|  |  |  |
|  |  |  |
|  |  |  |
|  |  |  |

# REFLECTION

# REFLECTION

# REFLECTION

REFLECTION

| DAYS | EXERCISES | CHECK |
|---|---|---|
|  |  |  |
|  |  |  |
|  |  |  |
|  |  |  |
|  |  |  |
|  |  |  |
|  |  |  |
|  |  |  |
|  |  |  |
|  |  |  |
|  |  |  |
|  |  |  |
|  |  |  |
|  |  |  |
|  |  |  |

# REFLECTION

# REFLECTION

# REFLECTION

REFLECTION

| DAYS | EXERCISES | CHECK |
| --- | --- | --- |
|  |  |  |
|  |  |  |
|  |  |  |
|  |  |  |
|  |  |  |
|  |  |  |
|  |  |  |
|  |  |  |
|  |  |  |
|  |  |  |
|  |  |  |
|  |  |  |
|  |  |  |
|  |  |  |

# REFLECTION

# REFLECTION

# REFLECTION

| DAYS | EXERCISES | CHECK |
|---|---|---|
|  |  |  |

# REFLECTION

# REFLECTION

# REFLECTION

# REFLECTION